# Simple Air Fryer Cookbook 2021

Simple Easy Delicious Recipes with your
Amazing Air Fryer and Keep on Enjoying
Healthy Meals

Martine Haley

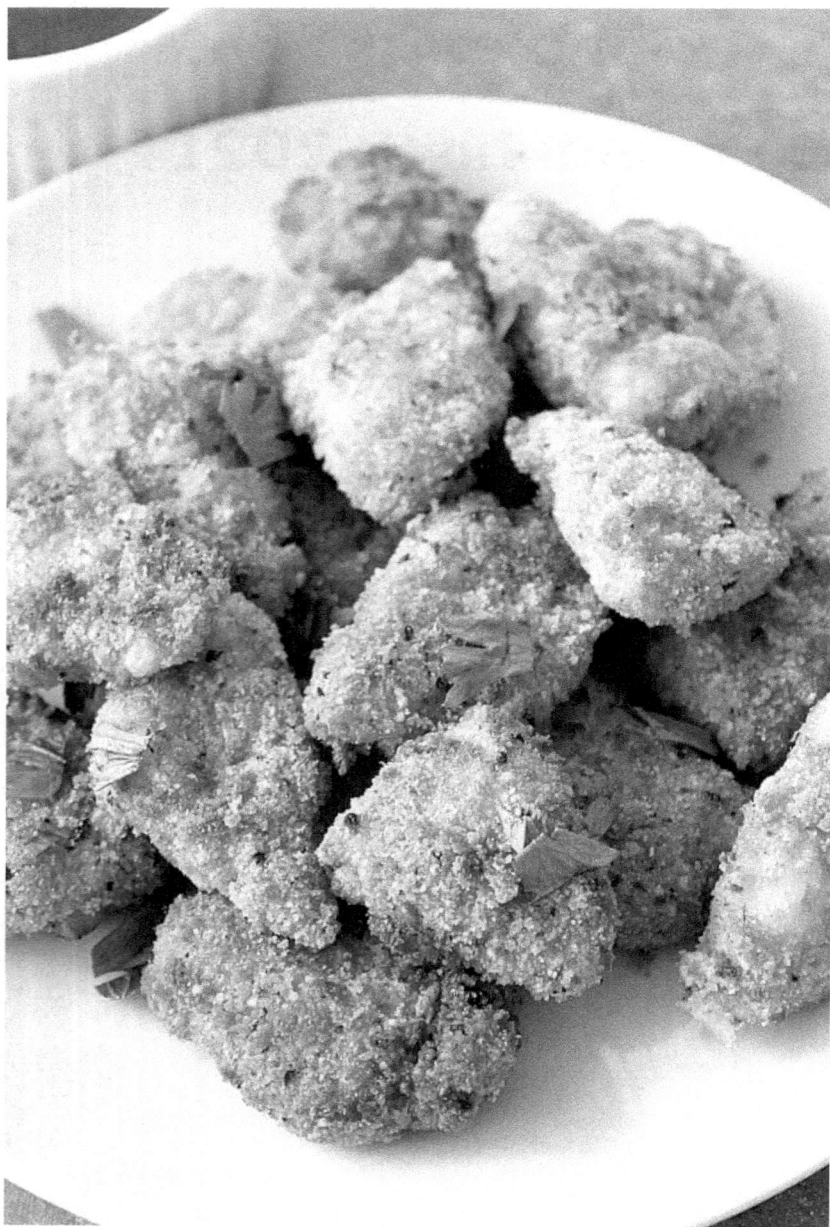

# Table of Contents

# INTRODUCTION

An air fryer is a kitchen appliance designed to deliver a tasty, crispy, golden-brown morsel of food without the use of oil or other cooking fats. It uses hot air instead of oil or other cooking fats to cook food quickly and evenly.

The air fryer can be used for making fried chips in addition to other foods.

There are several varieties of air fryers. One of the main categories is made up of countertop air fryers designed for individual use in the kitchen. These models sit on the worktop or counter top and feature a basket that sits on a wire rack. This forms the base that holds hot air that cooks food as it passes through it.

air fryer's air fryers are designed to help you make healthy and filling meals. Our electric fryers are perfect for people who want fresh, homemade fries without all of the fat. Our air fryer features a light-weight aluminum design that lets you move the appliance from room to room without worry. Each air fryer is also equipped with a thermostat, making it easy to adjust the temperature as needed.

An air fryer is an appliance that cooks food using high-speed air circulation. It is a perfect alternative to deep frying, baking or roasting, and works great for cooking fast and healthy meals.

How Does an Air Fryer Work?

The fan draws warm air from the bottom of the chamber, which rises and cools as it circulates. The food is then placed in the middle of the basket, and the fan circulates air around it, cooking it all at once. Food cooks faster than if you fried it in oil or baked it in an oven. The food doesn't become soggy like fried food does, either. Because the air circulates around the food rather than through it, you can use much less oil in your Air Fryer. Best of all, since no oil is being used for cooking, there's much less of an environmental impact!

What Types of Air Fryers are Available?

Air fryers come in a variety of sizes as well as different colors and designs. You may find one that has a View Master-like chrome trim or one with a retro design pattern that blends easily into your décor. Some Air fryers are as small as a rice cooker while others can be used to make large batches of French fries with recipes you create on your tablet! Some Air Fryer models have "smart" features that allow you to cook multiple foods at the same time; others have timers so you can automatically set them for particular times during the day. All versions sterilize their own cooking plates by running them through a clean cycle between batches!

When you are looking for a new air fryer, you should take a look at air fryer Cookware. We have all of the features you are looking for in an air fryer, including built in racks that will allow you to cook a full size meal for your family. We also have a variety of accessories that will give you an even better cooking experience.

We are proud to introduce air fryer Cookware, the premier brand in air fryers. You can rest assured that we only use the best materials to ensure our products will work for years to come. Our air fryers feature built-in racks, so you can cook a full-size meal at once. They also include an adjustable thermostat that ranges from 120 to 500 degrees Fahrenheit.

Whether you are looking to impress your family with gourmet French fries or just want to make your favorite chicken drumsticks and vegetables, air fryer Cookware has everything you need. Every item has been carefully tested to ensure safe and responsible use. All of our products carry a One Year Limited Manufacturer Warranty, so you can be confident that they will serve your needs well.

# BREAKFAST

## Sausage and Cream Cheese Biscuits

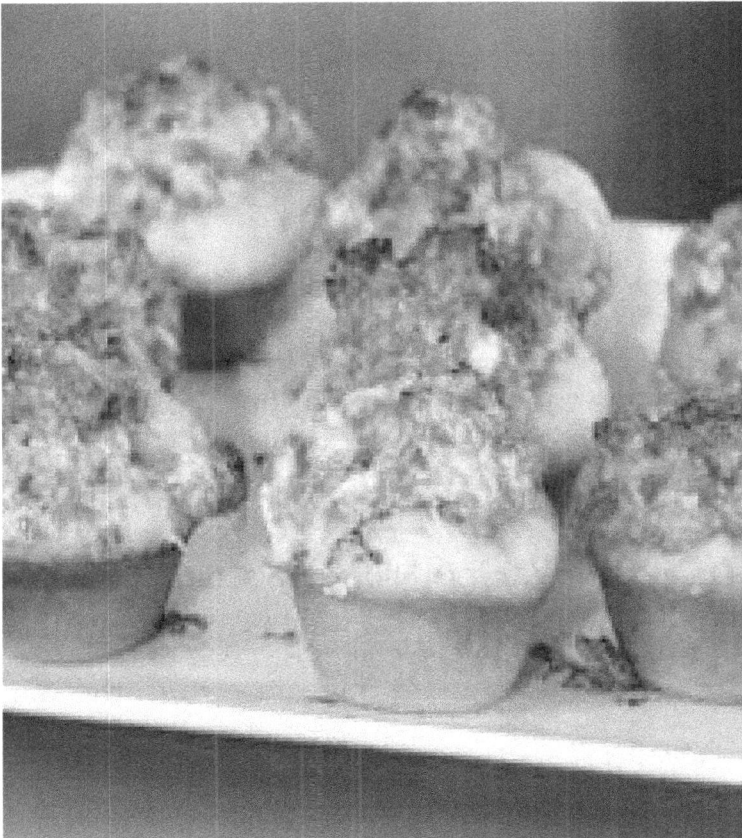

Preparation Time: 5 Minutes

Cooking Time: 15 Minutes

Servings: 5

**Ingredients:**

- 12 ounces chicken breakfast sausage
- 1 (6-ounce) can biscuits
- ⅛ Cup cream cheese

**Directions:**

1. Form the sausage into 5 small patties.
2. Place the sausage patties in the air fryer. Cook for 5 minutes.
3. Open the air fryer. Flip the patties. Cook for an additional 5 minutes.
4. Remove the cooked sausages from the air fryer.
5. Separate the biscuit dough into 5 biscuits.
6. Place the biscuits in the air fryer. Cook for 3 minutes.
7. Open the air fryer. Flip the biscuits. Cook for an additional 2 minutes.
8. Remove the cooked biscuits from the air fryer.
9. Split each biscuit in half. Spread 1 teaspoon of cream cheese onto the bottom of each biscuit. Top with a sausage patty and the other half of the biscuit, and serve.

**Nutrition:** Calories: 249 Total fat: 13g Saturated fat: 7g Cholesterol: 6mg Sodium: 556mg Carbohydrates: 20g Fiber: 0g Protein: 9g

# Breakfast Grilled Ham and Cheese

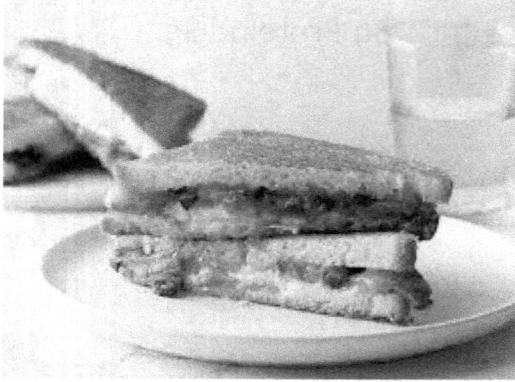

Preparation Time: 5 Minutes

Cooking Time: 10 Minutes

Servings: 2

**Ingredients:**

- 1 teaspoon butter
- 4 slices bread
- 4 slices smoked country ham
- 4 slices Cheddar cheese
- 4 thick slices tomato

**Directions:**

1. Spread ½ teaspoon of butter onto one side of 2 slices of bread. Each sandwich will have 1 slice of bread with butter and 1 slice without.
2. Assemble each sandwich by layering 2 slices of ham, 2 slices of cheese, and 2 slices of

tomato on the unbuttered pieces of bread. Put it on top of the other bread slices, with the buttered side up.

3. Place the sandwiches in the air fryer buttered-side down. Cook for 4 minutes.

4. Open the air fryer. Flip the grilled cheese sandwiches. Cook for an additional 4 minutes.

5. Cool before serving. Cut each sandwich in half and enjoy.

**Nutrition:** Calories: 525 Total fat: 25g Saturated fat: 14g Cholesterol: 88mg Sodium: 1618mg Carbohydrates: 34g Fiber: 5g Protein: 41g

# Classic Hash Browns

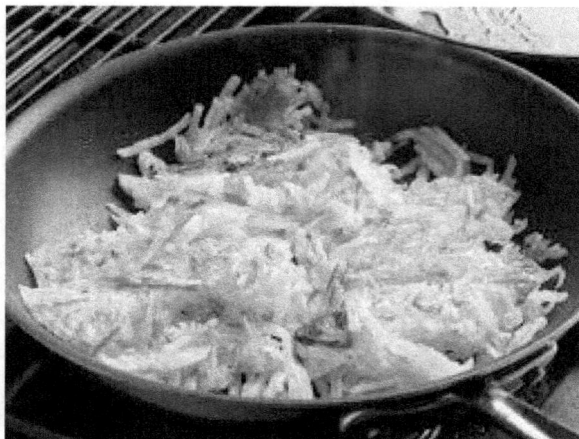

Preparation Time: 15 Minutes

Cooking Time: 20 Minutes

Servings: 4

**Ingredients:**

- 4 russet potatoes
- 1 teaspoon paprika
- Salt
- Pepper
- Cooking oil

**Directions:**

1. Peel the potatoes using a vegetable peeler. Using a cheese grater, shred the potatoes. If your grater has different-size holes, use the area of the tool with the largest holes.

2. Place the grated potatoes in a large bowl with cold water. Let it sit for 5 minutes. Cold water helps remove excess starch from the potatoes. Stir to help dissolve the starch.
3. Drain the potatoes and dry with paper towels or napkins. Make sure the potatoes are completely dry.
4. Season the potatoes with the paprika and salt and pepper to taste.
5. Spray the potatoes with cooking oil and transfer them to the air fryer. Cook for 20 minutes, moving the basket every 5 minutes (a total of 4 times).
6. Cool before serving.

**Nutrition:** Calories: 150 Total fat: 0g Saturated fat: 0g Cholesterol: 0mg Sodium: 52mg Carbohydrates: 34g Fiber: 5g Protein: 4g

# Canadian Bacon and Cheese English Muffins

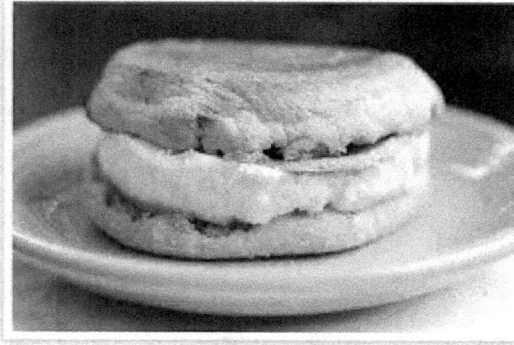

Preparation Time: 5 Minutes

Cooking Time: 10 Minutes

Servings: 4

**Ingredients:**

- 4 English muffins
- 8 slices Canadian bacon
- 4 slices cheese
- Cooking oil

**Directions:**

1. Split each English muffin. Assemble the breakfast sandwiches by layering 2 slices of Canadian bacon and 1 slice of cheese onto each English muffin bottom. Put it on top of the other half of the English muffin.

2. Place the sandwiches in the air fryer. Spray the top of each with cooking oil. Cook for 4 minutes.

3. Open the air fryer and flip the sandwiches. Cook for an additional 4 minutes.

4. Cool before serving.

**Nutrition:** Calories: 333 Total fat: 14g Saturated fat: 8g Cholesterol: 58mg Sodium: 1219mg Carbohydrates: 27g Fiber: 2g Protein: 24g

# Avocado Taco Fry

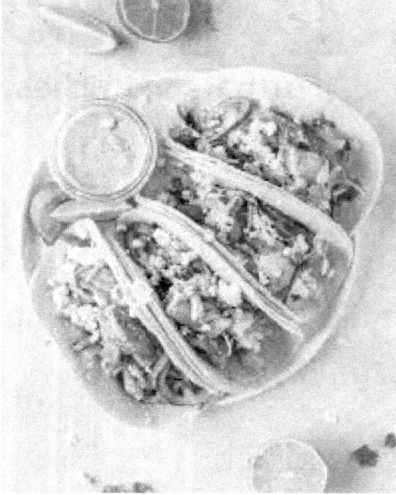

Preparation Time: 5 minutes

Cooking Time: 20 minutes

Servings: 12 slices

## Ingredients:

- 1 peeled avocado, sliced
- 1 beaten egg
- 1/2 cup panko bread crumbs
- Salt
- Tortillas and toppings

## Directions:

1. Using a bowl, add in the egg.
2. Using a separate bowl, set in the breadcrumbs.

3. Dip the avocado into the bowl with the beaten egg and coat with the breadcrumbs. Sprinkle the coated wedges with a bit of salt.
4. Arrange them in the cooking basket in a single layer.
5. Set the Air Fryer to 392 degrees and cook for 15 minutes. Shake the basket halfway through the cooking process.
6. Put them on tortillas with your preferred toppings.

**Nutrition:** Calorie: 140 kcal Carbs: 12g Fat: 8.8g Protein: 6g

# Cinnamon and Cheese Pancake

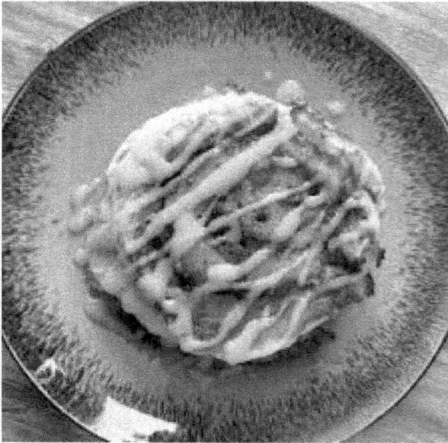

Preparation Time: 7 minutes

Cooking Time: 20 minutes

Servings: 4

**Ingredients:**

- 2 eggs
- 2 cups reduced-fat cream cheese
- 1/2 tsp. cinnamon
- 1 pack Stevia

**Directions:**

1. Adjust the Air Fryer to 330ºF.
2. In a blender, mix cream cheese, cinnamon, eggs, and stevia.
3. Pour a quarter of the mixture into the Air fryer basket. Cook for 2 minutes on all sides.

Repeat the process with the remaining portion of the mixture. Serve.

**Nutrition:** Calories: 140 kcal Carbs: 5.4g Fat: 10.6g Protein: 22.7g

# Scallion Sandwich

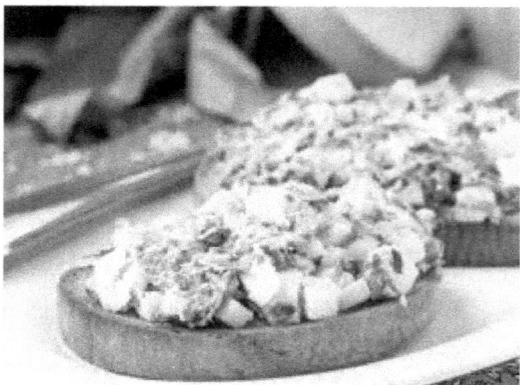

Preparation Time: 10 minutes

Cooking Time: 15 minutes

Servings: 1

**Ingredients:**

- 2 slices wheat bread
- 2 tsps. Low-fat butter
- 2 sliced scallions
- 1 tbsp. grated parmesan cheese
- 3/4 cup low-fat, grated cheddar cheese

**Directions:**

1. Adjust the Air fryer to 356ºF.
2. Apply butter to a slice of bread. Then place it inside the cooking basket with the butter side facing down.

3. Place cheese and scallions on top. Spread the rest of the butter on the other slice of bread. Then put it on top of the sandwich and sprinkle with parmesan cheese.
4. Allow to cook for 10 minutes. Serve.

**Nutrition:** Calories: 154 kcal Carbs: 9g Fat: 2.5g Protein: 8.6g

# Cinnamon Pancake

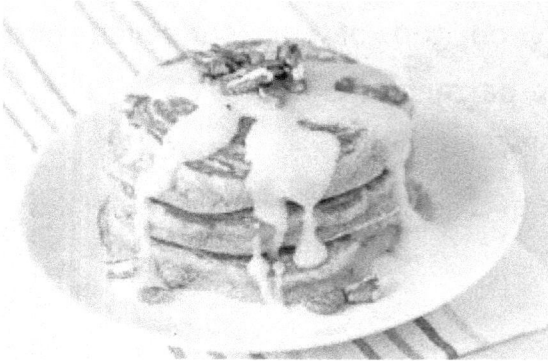

Preparation Time: 15 minutes

Cooking Time: 20 minutes

Servings: 4

**Ingredients:**

- 2 eggs
- 2 cups low-fat cream cheese
- 1/2 tsp. cinnamon
- 1 pack Stevia

**Directions:**

1. Adjust the temp. to 330ºF.
2. Combine cream cheese, cinnamon, eggs, and stevia in a blender.
3. Pour a quarter of the mixture in the air fryer basket.
4. Allow to cook for 2 minutes on both sides.

5. Repeat the process with the rest of the mixture. Serve.

**Nutrition:** Calories: 106 kcal Carbs: 10g Fat: 3.2g Protein: 9g

# Fried Egg

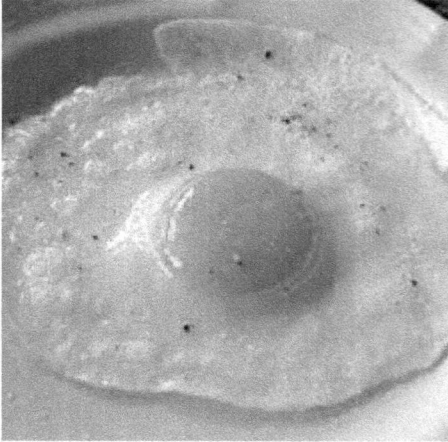

Preparation Time: 5 minutes

Cooking Time: 4 minutes

Servings: 1

**Ingredients:**

- 1 pastured egg
- 1/8 tsp. salt
- 1/8 tbsp. cracked black pepper

**Directions:**

1. Grease the fryer pan with olive oil then crack the egg in it.
2. Insert the fryer pan into the air fryer, close the lid. Then adjust the fryer to 370ºF.

3. After 3minutes, open the air fryer to check if the egg needs more cooking. If yes, leave it for an extra 1 minute.

4. Serve the egg. Add salt and black pepper to season it.

**Nutrition:** Calories: 90 kcal Carbs: 0.6 g Fat: 7 g Protein: 6.3 g

# Air Fryer Scrambled Egg

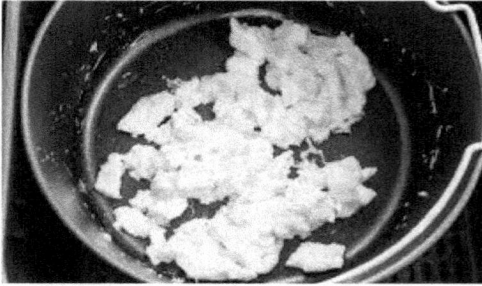

Preparation Time: 5 minutes

Cooking Time: 10 minutes

Servings: 2

**Ingredients:**

- 2 eggs
- 1 chopped tomato
- Dash of salt
- 1 tsp. butter
- 1/4 cup cream

**Directions:**

1. Put the eggs in a bowl then add salt and the cream. Whisk until fluffy.
2. Adjust the air fryer to 300°F.
3. Add butter to baking pan and place it into the preheated air fryer.
4. Add the egg mixture to the baking pan once the butter has melted.

5. Cook for 10-minutes. Serve warm.

**Nutrition:** Calories: 105 kcal Carbs: 2.3g Fat:  8g Protein:  6.4g

# Breakfast Cheese Bread Cups

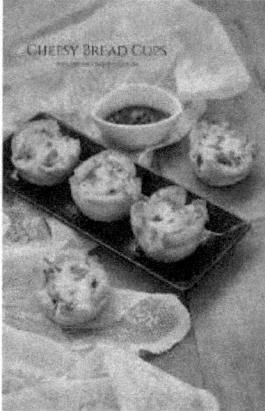

Preparation Time: 6 minutes

Cooking Time: 15 minutes

Servings: 2

**Ingredients:**

- 2 eggs
- 2 tbsps. Grated cheddar cheese
- Salt and pepper
- 1 ham slice cut into 2 pieces
- 4 bread slices flatted with a rolling pin

**Directions:**

1. Spray both sides of the ramekins with cooking spray.
2. Place two slices of bread into each ramekin.
3. Add the ham slice pieces into each ramekin.

4. Crack an egg in each ramekin then sprinkle with cheese.
5. Season with salt and pepper.
6. Place the ramekins into air fryer at 300°Fahrenheit for 15-minutes.
7. Serve warm.

**Nutrition:** Calories: 162 kcal Total Fat: 8g Carbs: 10g Protein: 11g

# Cheese & Egg Breakfast Sandwich

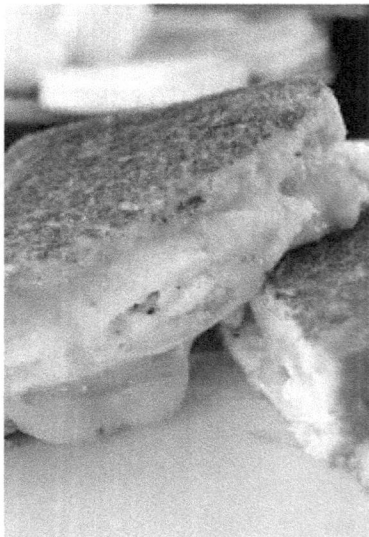

Preparation Time: 3 minutes

Cooking Time: 6 minutes

Servings: 1

**Ingredients:**

- 1 egg
- 2 slices cheddar or Swiss cheese
- A bit of butter
- 1 roll either English muffin or Kaiser Bun, halved

**Directions:**

1. Butter the sliced rolls on both sides.
2. Whisk the eggs in an oven-safe dish.

3. Place the cheese, egg dish, and rolls into the air fryer. Make sure the buttered sides of the roll are facing upwards.

4. Adjust the air fryer to 390°F. Cook for 6 minutes.

5. Place the egg and cheese between the pieces of roll. Serve warm.

**Nutrition:** Calories: 212 kcal Total Fat: 11.2g Carbs: 9.3g Protein: 12.4g

# Peanut Butter & Banana Breakfast Sandwich

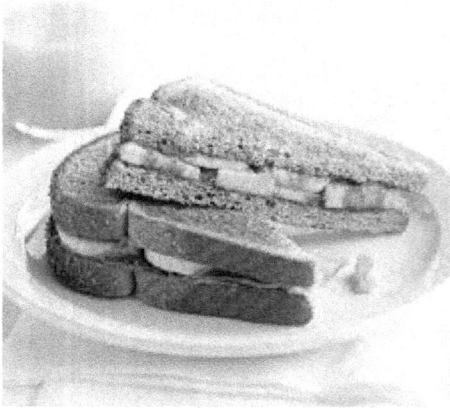

Preparation Time: 4 minutes

Cooking Time: 6 minutes

Servings: 1

**Ingredients:**

- 2 slices whole-wheat bread
- 1 tsp. sugar-free maple syrup
- 1 sliced banana
- 2 tbsps. Peanut butter

**Directions:**

1. Evenly coat each side of the sliced bread with peanut butter.

2. Add the sliced banana and drizzle with some sugar-free maple syrup.

3. Adjust the air fryer to 330°F then cook for 6 minutes. Serve warm.

**Nutrition:** Calories: 211 kcal Total Fat: 8.2g Carbs: 6.3g Protein: 11.2g

# Breakfast Frittata

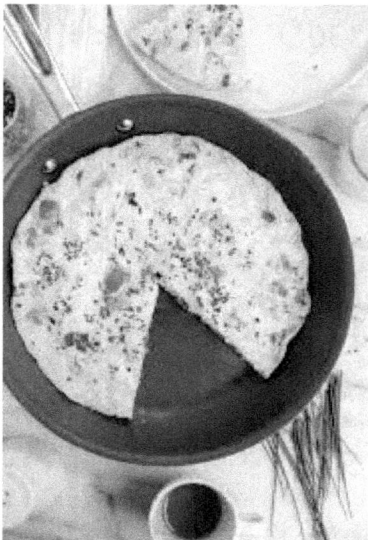

Preparation Time: 5 minutes

Cooking Time: 15 minutes

Servings: 3

## Ingredients:

- 6 eggs
- 8 halved cherry tomatoes
- 2 tbsps. shredded parmesan cheese
- 1 Italian sausage, diced
- Salt and pepper

## Directions:

1. Adjust the air fryer to 355°F.

2. Add the tomatoes and sausage to the baking dish.

3. Place the baking dish into the air fryer and cook for 5 minutes.

4. Meanwhile, add eggs, cheese, salt, oil, and pepper into mixing bowl then whisk properly.

5. Remove the baking dish from the air fryer and pour the egg mixture on top. Ensure you spread it evenly.

6. Place the dish back into the air fryer and bake for an additional 5 minutes.

7. Remove from air fryer and slice into wedges and serve.

**Nutrition:** Calories: 273 kcal Total Fat: 8.2g Carbs: 7g Protein: 14.2g

# Morning Mini Cheeseburger Sliders

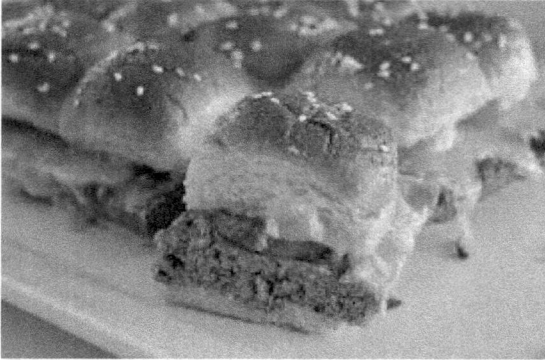

Preparation Time: 5 minutes

Cooking Time: 10 minutes

Servings: 6

**Ingredients:**

- 1 lb. ground beef
- 6 slices cheddar cheese
- 6 dinner rolls
- Salt and Black pepper

**Directions:**

Adjust the air fryer to 390°F.

1. Form 6 beef patties (each about 2.5 oz.) and season with salt and black pepper.
2. Add the burger patties to the cooking basket and cook them for 10 minutes.

3. Remove the burger patties from the air fryer; place the cheese on top of burgers and return to the air fryer and cook for another minute.
4. Remove and put burgers on dinner rolls and serve warm.

**Nutrition:** Calories: 262 kcal Total Fat: 9.4g Carbs: 8.2g Protein: 16.2g

# Grilled Cheese

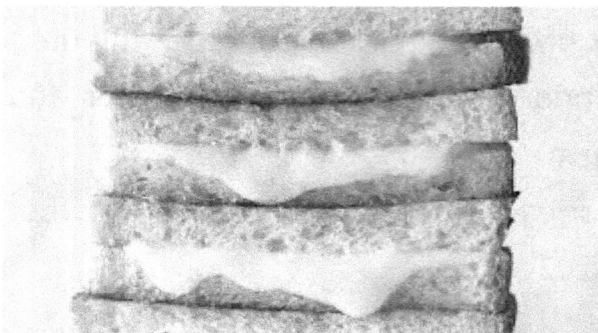

Preparation Time: 4 minutes

Cooking Time: 7 minutes

Servings: 2

**Ingredients:**

- 4 slices brown bread
- 1/2 cup shredded sharp cheddar cheese
- 1/4 cup melted butter

**Directions:**

1. Adjust your air fryer to 360°F.
2. In separate bowls, place cheese and butter.
3. Melt butter and brush it onto the 4 slices of bread.
4. Place cheese on 2 sides of bread slices.
5. Put sandwiches together and place them into the cooking basket.
6. Cook for 5 minutes and serve warm.

**Nutrition:** Calories: 214 kcal Total Fat: 11.2g Carbs: 9.4g Protein: 13.2g

# Breakfast Muffins

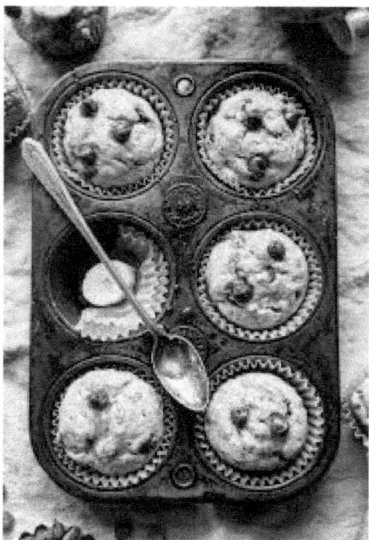

Preparation Time: 3 minutes

Cooking Time: 6 minutes

Servings: 2

**Ingredients:**

- 2 whole-wheat English muffins
- 4 slices bacon
- Pepper
- 2 eggs

**Directions:**

1. Crack an egg each into ramekins then season with pepper.

2. Place the ramekins in your preheated air fryer at 390°F.

3. Allow to cock for 6-minutes with the bacon and muffins alongside.

4. Remove the muffins from the air fryer after a few minutes and split them.

5. When the bacon and eggs are done cooking, add two pieces of bacon and one egg to each egg muffin. Serve when hot.

**Nutrition:** Calories: 276 kcal Total Fat: 12g Carbs: 10.2g Protein: 17.3g

# Bacon BBQ

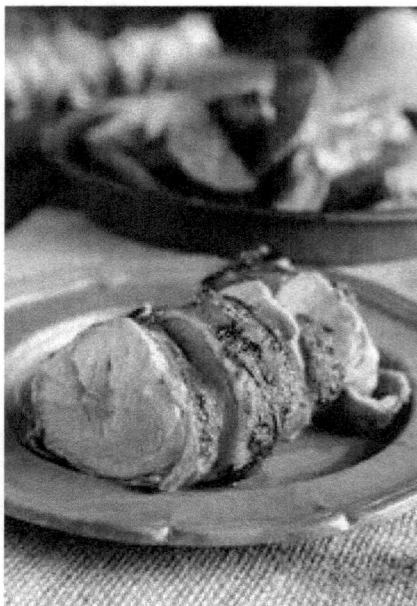

Preparation Time: 2 minutes

Cooking Time: 8 minutes

Servings: 2

**Ingredients:**

- 13g dark brown sugar
- 5g chili powder
- 1g ground cumin
- 1g cayenne pepper
- 4 slices bacon, halved

**Directions:**

1. Mix seasonings until well combined.

2. Dip the bacon in the dressing until it is completely covered. Leave aside.

3. Adjust the air fryer to 160°C.

4. Place the bacon in the preheated air fryer

5. Select Bacon option and press Start/Pause. Serve.

**Nutrition:** Calories: 1124 kcal Fat: 72g Carbs: 59g Protein: 49g

# Crashed Bones with Chips and Ham

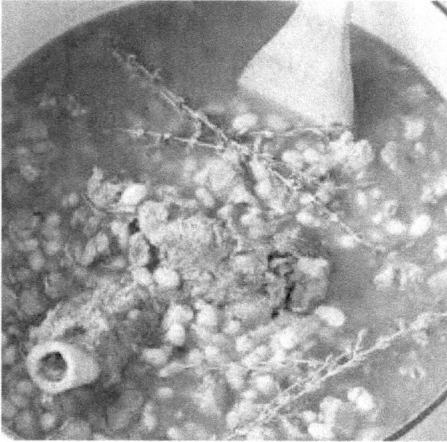

Preparation Time: 5 minutes

Cooking Time: 20 minutes

Servings: 4

**Ingredients:**

- 600g potatoes
- Salt
- 1 tbsp olive oil
- 100g Iberian Ham
- 4 eggs

**Directions:**

1. Cut the elongated French fries, rinse through plenty of water and dry well with paper towels.
2. Spray with oil and adjust the air fryer to 200°C for a few minutes.
3. Put the potatoes in the air fryer and set the timer for 25 minutes at 200°C.
4. When we see that they are starting to brown, put paper under the potatoes, and lay the eggs.
5. Put in the air fryer again 5 more minutes.
6. Finally, add Iberian ham flakes.
7. If you want to go faster while the potatoes are fried in the air fryer, you can prepare the grilled eggs in a small pan and then mix with the potatoes and ham on the plate. Serve.

**Nutrition:** Calories: 162.6 kcal Fat: 12g Carbs: 0.6g Protein: 16.6g

# French Toast Sticks

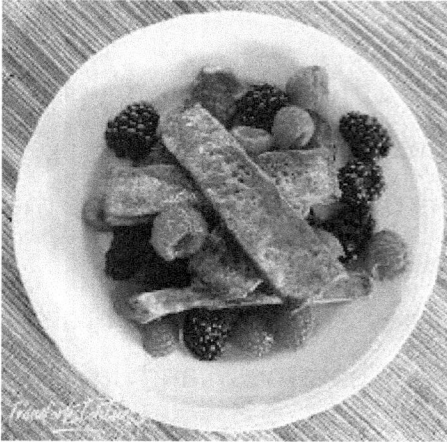

Preparation Time: 5 Minutes

Cooking Time: 10 Minutes

Servings: 2

**Ingredients:**

- 2 eggs
- 1/4 cup whole milk
- 1/4 cup brown sugar
- 4 slices whole meal bread
- 1 teaspoon cinnamon or nutmeg

**Directions:**

1. Cut each piece of bread vertically into 4 identical strips.
2. Beat the eggs in a large bowl, then add all other ingredients together in the same bowl.

3. Dip each bread strip into the bowl then drip off the excess batter.

4. Preheat the fryer to 360 and place all the strips in the basket.

5. Cook for 10 minutes, flipping them over at the halfway point.

**Nutrition:** Calories: 348 Sodium: 79 mg Dietary Fiber: 6g Fat: 6.9g Carbs: 56.4g Protein: 15g.

# Ham and Egg Toast Cups

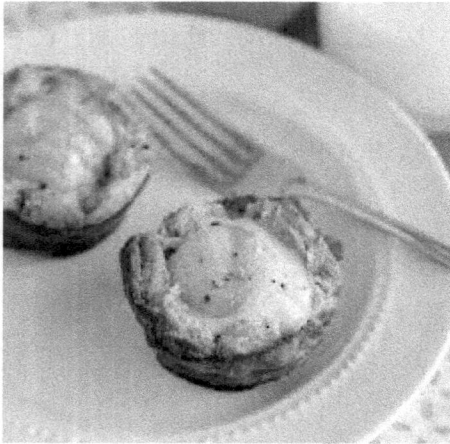

Preparation Time: 10 Minutes

Cooking Time: 15 Minutes

Servings: 2

**Ingredients:**

- 2 eggs
- 4 slices of bread
- 1 slice of ham
- Melted butter
- Salt and pepper to taste

**Directions:**

1. Grease the inside of the ramekin with melted butter.
2. Toast bread and flatten it with a rolling pin.

3. Press 1 piece of toast into the bottom of the ramekin to create a bread bowl.
4. Press another piece of toast onto the first one to create a double layer.
5. Cut the ham into 4 slices then line the inside of the toast cups with 2 strips of ham each.
6. Crack an egg into the middle of each cup and season with salt and pepper.
7. Cook it in the air fryer for 15 minutes at 320 degrees, if you like your eggs less runny, you may want to add a few minutes to the cook time.

**Nutrition:** Calories: 202 Sodium: 488 mg Dietary Fiber: 1.6 g Fat: 2.6 g Carbs: 16 g Protein: 9.2 g.

# Air Fryer Sausage Wraps

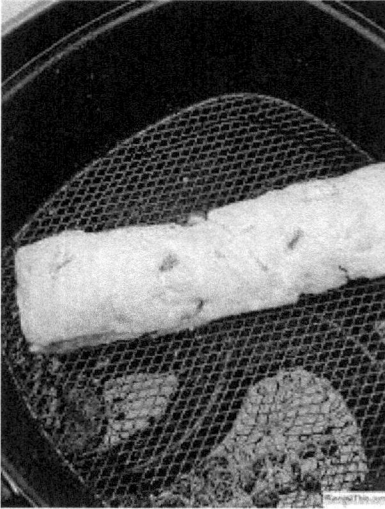

Preparation Time: 5 Minutes

Cooking Time: 3 Minutes

Servings: 2

**Ingredients:**

- 8 pre-cooked sausages
- 2 pieces American cheese
- 1 can of 8 count refrigerated crescent roll dough

**Directions:**

1. Cut each of the cheese slices into corners.
2. Unroll eat crescent roll.
3. At the wide end of the crescent roll, put down 1/4 of cheese and 1 sausage.

4. Starting at the wide end, roll the crescent up and tuck in the ends to cover the sausage and cheese.
5. Preheat the fryer to 380 degrees.
6. Put them in the basket and cook for about 3 minutes.

**Nutrition:** Calories: 325 Sodium: 783 mg Dietary Fiber: 0.5g Fat: 24.7g Carbs: 7.9 g Protein: 16.7 g.

# Bacon Egg and Cheese Eggroll

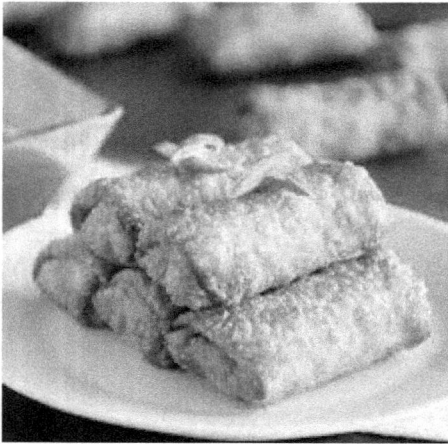

Preparation Time: 15 Minutes

Cooking Time: 10 Minutes

Servings: 5

**Ingredients:**

- 4 eggs
- 4 slices bacon
- 1/2 cup shredded cheddar cheese
- 5 egg roll wrappers

**Directions:**

1. In a big pan, fry the bacon until crispy and set aside.
2. Drain the bacon fat, but leave a little left behind in the skillet.
3. Using the bacon fat, scramble your eggs.

4. Roll out your eggroll wrappers.

5. In a separate bowl, crumble, the bacon into tiny pieces, then mix in the eggs and the cheese.

6. Scoop in equal amounts of the mixture to the center of each wrapper.

7. Pull the bottom left corner of the wrapper over the mixture, then fold each side in.

8. Wet the remaining edge and roll the eggroll shut.

9. Preheat the air fryer to 360 degrees and cook for 10 minutes flipping eggrolls halfway through.

**Nutrition:** Calories: 302 Sodium: 483 mg Dietary Fiber: 0.6g Fat: 18.5g Carbs: 19.2 g Protein: 13.8g.

# Air Fryer Breakfast Potatoes

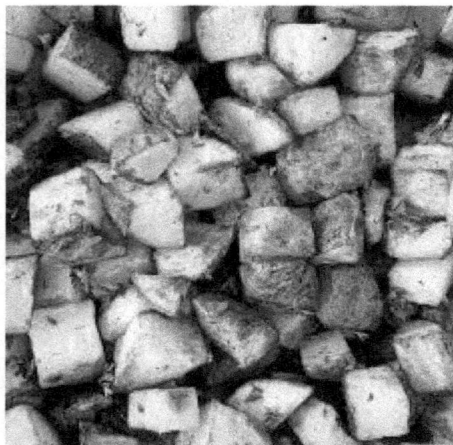

Preparation Time: 10 Minutes

Cooking Time: 25 Minutes

Servings: 4

**Ingredients:**

- 2 russet potatoes
- 1 red bell pepper
- 1 white onion
- Cooking spray
- Salt and pepper to taste

**Directions:**

1. Cut the potatoes into 1-inch small cubes.
2. Put them in the basket, spray with cooking spray, and sprinkle with a little salt and pepper.

3. Cook the potatoes at 400 degrees for 10 minutes, shaking once at the halfway point.

4. While the potatoes cook dice up the peppers and onions into small cubes.

5. Mix in the onions and peppers with the potatoes. Season with salt and pepper.

6. Cook at 400 for another 15 minutes shaking a few times and checking to make sure that the potatoes aren't being overcooked.

**Nutrition:** Calories: 376 Sodium: 33 mg Dietary Fiber: 14.2g Fat: 0.8g Carbs: 86.2 g Protein: 9.6g.

# Chocolate Filled Donut Holes

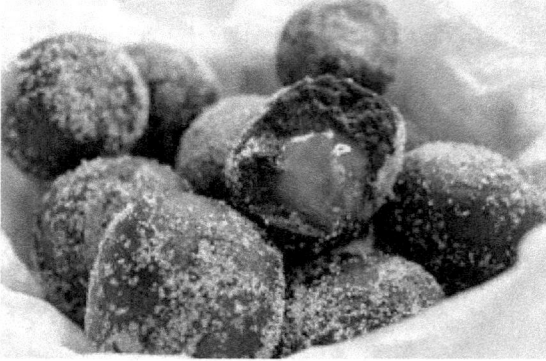

Preparation Time: 10 Minutes

Cooking Time: 12 Minutes

Servings: 6

**Ingredients:**

- 1 (8-count) can refrigerated biscuits
- 1 bag semi-sweet chocolate chips
- 3 tablespoons melted butter
- 1/4 cup powdered sugar

**Directions:**

1. Cut each biscuit on into thirds.
2. Flatten each third with your hands and put a small dimple in the center with your thumb.
3. Place 2 – 3 chocolate chips inside each dimple and wrap the dough around the chocolate chips creating a ball.

4. Brush each ball with butter.

5. Cook at 320 for 10 minutes tossing at least once to ensure even baking throughout.

6. Place powdered sugar in bowl.

7. As soon as your donut holes are done put them in the powdered sugar and toss before serving.

**Nutrition:** Calories: 297 Sodium: 705 mg Dietary Fiber: 0.6g Fat: 15.5g Carbs: 35.4 g Protein: 4.7g.

# All in One Breakfast Sandwich

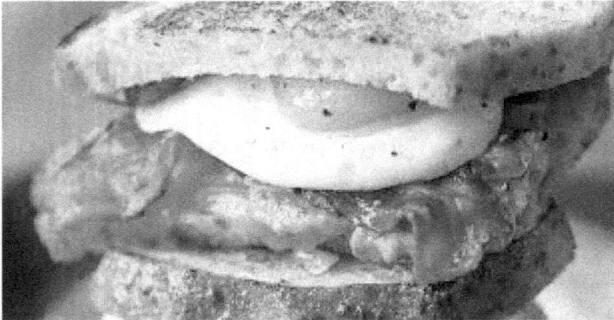

Preparation Time: 1 Minute

Cooking Time: 6 Minutes

Servings: 1

**Ingredients:**

- 1 egg
- 1 English muffin
- 2 pieces bacon
- 1 slice cheddar cheese
- Salt and pepper to taste

**Directions:**

1. Break egg in the ramekin and add salt and pepper.
2. Preheat the air fryer to 400.
3. Place all the ingredients (expect for the cheese) in the basket separately and cook for 5 minutes.

4. Assemble the sandwich with the bottom of the muffin, the egg, the cheese, the bacon, and the top of the muffin in that order.

**Nutrition:** Calories: 404 Sodium: 745 mg Dietary Fiber: 3.3g Fat: 21.6g Carbs: 32.5 g Protein: 18.6g.

# Banana Bites

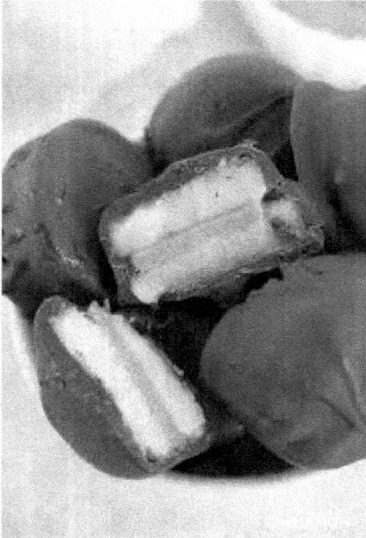

Preparation Time: 10 Minutes

Cooking Time: 10 Minutes

Servings: 6

**Ingredients:**

- 3 bananas
- 1 cup dry pancake mix
- 1 cup milk
- 1 egg
- 1 teaspoon vanilla

**Directions:**

1. Combine the egg, milk, vanilla, and pancake mix in a medium bowl.

2. Cut every single banana into 1/2-inch slices.

3. Use a fork to dip each banana slice in the pancake mix allowing extra batter to drip off.

4. Cook in your basket at 320 degrees for 10 minutes, tossing 1 or 2 times.

5. Serve with a side of maple syrup for dipping.

**Nutrition:** Calories: 114 Sodium: 60 mg Dietary Fiber: 1.6g Fat: 1.9g Carbs: 22.3g Protein: 3.1g.

# Sausage Balls

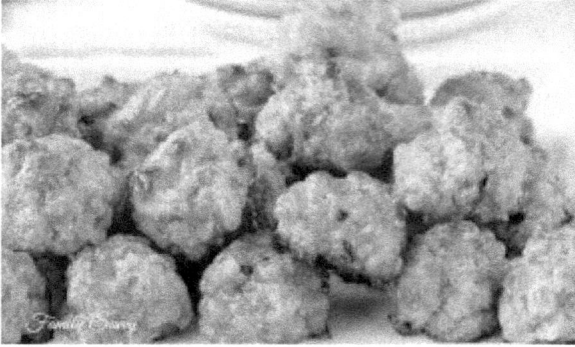

Preparation Time: 10 Minutes

Cooking Time: 20 Minutes

Servings: 10

**Ingredients:**

- 1-pound breakfast sausage
- 1 egg
- 1 cup almond meal
- 1 cup sharp cheddar cheese
- 2 teaspoons baking powder

**Directions:**

1. Put all of the ingredients in a bowl and mix it well. Considering the consistency of these ingredients, you may want to use and electric mixer to save your shoulders.
2. Preheat your fryer to 350 degrees.

3. Spoon out small scoops and roll them into balls and place them in your basket giving them room to breathe. This recipe makes about 30 balls, so you will probably have to do at least 2 batches.

4. Cook for 350 minutes, tossing at the 10- and 15-minute mark.

**Nutrition:** Calories: 262 Sodium: 533 mg Dietary Fiber: 1.2g Fat: 21.8g Carbs: 2.7g Protein: 14.2g.

# Bacon

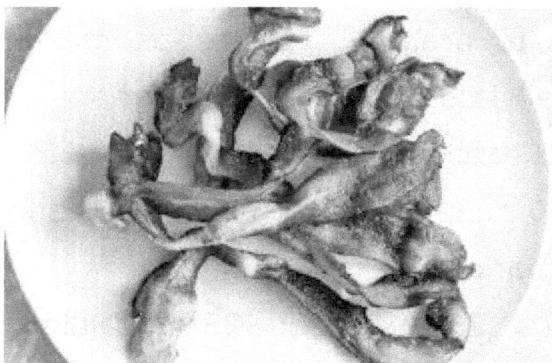

Preparation Time: 11 minutes

Cooking Time: 11 minutes

Servings: 8 to 11 people

**Ingredients:**

- 11 slices of bacon

**Directions:**

1. Divide all of the bacon in half, and put the first half in the Air Fryer and cook for about 5 to 10 minutes depending on the size of the bacon at 4000F.

2. Check it after 5 minutes of cooking to see if anything needs to be rearranged using tongs.

3. Cook for the remaining time and check for desired doneness for about 1.5 minutes extra for a total of 11.5 minutes.

**Nutrition:** Calories: 80 Protein: 5 g Fat: 7 g Carbs: 1 g

# Bacon and Brown Sugar Little Smokies

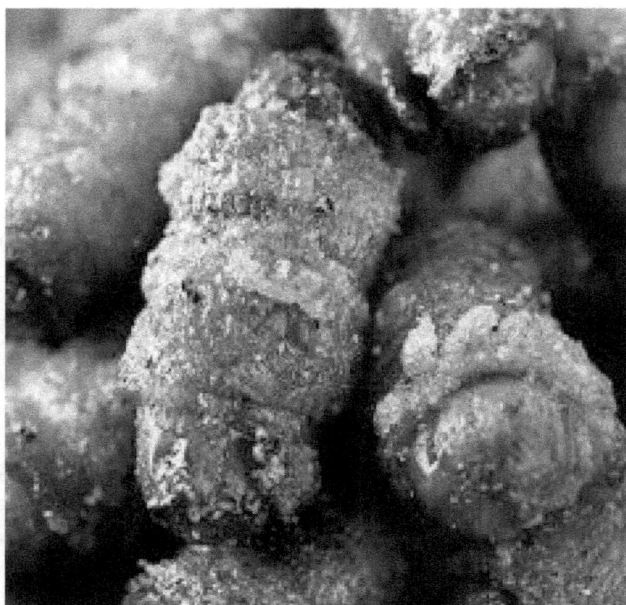

Preparation Time: 10 minutes

Cooking Time: 10 minutes

Servings: 6 to 8 people

**Ingredients:**

- 14 ounces of Little Smokies
- 2/3 ounce of Bacon
- 1/3 cup of Brown Sugar Substitute
- Toothpicks

**Directions:**

1. Cut Bacon tips into thirds, and put the brown sugar substitute into a shallow dish that is enough to fit the bacon thirds.
2. Place a slice of bacon into the brown sugar substitute and coat on both sides.
3. Wrap one little smokie by a slice of brown sugar-coated bacon and pin it with a Toothpick.
4. Repeat with the rest of the little smokies and then place them inside of the Air fryer basket.
5. Cook at 3500F for about 10 minutes until the bacon is crisped, flip halfway through the cooking process.

**Nutrition:** Calories: 680 Carbs: 41 g Fat: 27 g Protein: 15 g

# Hard Eggs

Preparation Time: 1 minute

Cooking Time: 15 minutes

Servings: 4-6

**Ingredients:**

- 1-6 large eggs

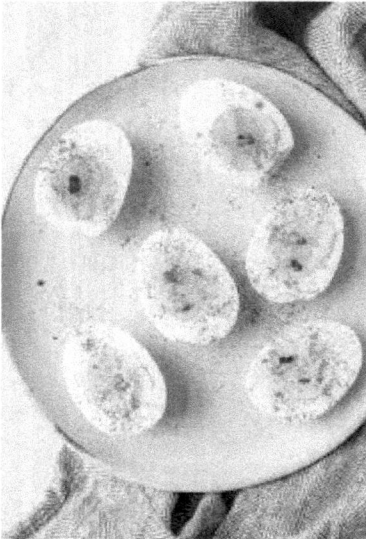

**Directions:**

1. Preheat Air fryer to 2700F after that place eggs in Air fryer basket and cook on 2700F for about 15 minutes.

2. Once timer is done, remove from Air fryer basket and place in bowl filled with ice water for 5 minutes.

3. Remove and peel.

**Nutrition:** Calories: 80 Carbs: 1 g Fat: 2 g Protein: 5 g

# Morning Sandwich Cheesy Stuffed

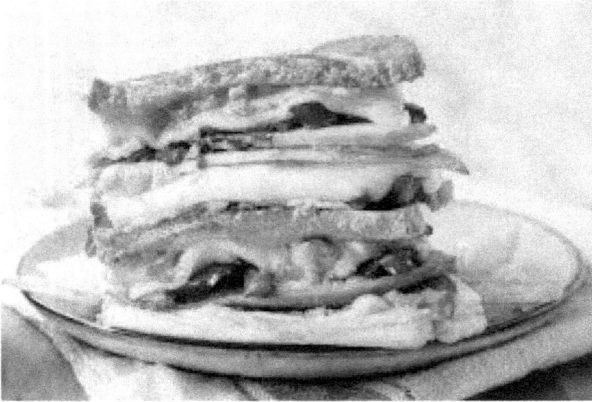

Preparation Time: 1 minute

Cooking Time: 8 minutes

Servings: 2

**Ingredients:**

- 1 tbsp. butter
- 4 frozen bread slices
- 2 cheddar cheese slices

**Directions:**

1. Evenly spread butter on each bread slice evenly.
2. Place one cheese slice between two bread slices.
3. Preheat your Air Fryer to a temperature of 360°F.

4. Transfer sandwiches into fryer basket and let them cook for 8 minutes.

5. Serve with coffee or tea, or with vegetables.

**Nutrition:** Calories: 272    Protein: 10.39 g Fat: 16.56 g Carbs: 20.37 g

# Grilled Ham and Cheese

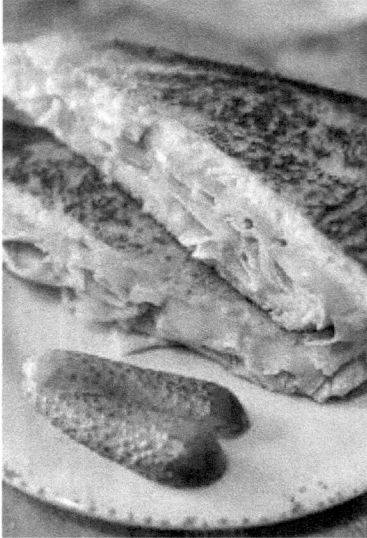

Preparation Time: 5 minutes

Cooking Time: 10 minutes

Servings: 2

**Ingredients:**

- 4 slices smoked country ham
- 4 slices bread
- 4 thick slices tomato
- 1 tsp. butter
- 4 slices Cheddar cheese

**Directions:**

1. Spread ½ tsp. of butter onto one side of 2 slices of bread. Each sandwich will have 1 slice of bread with butter and 1 slice without.
2. Assemble each sandwich by layering 2 slices of ham, 2 slices of cheese, and 2 slices of tomato on the unbuttered pieces of bread. Put it on top of the rest of the bread slices, with the buttered side up.
3. Place the sandwiches in53 the air fryer buttered-side down. Cook for 4 minutes.
4. Open the air fryer. Flip the grilled cheese sandwiches. Cook for an additional 4 minutes.
5. Cool before serving.
6. Cut each sandwich in half and enjoy.

**Nutrition:** Calories: 525 Fat: 25g Carbs: 34g Protein: 41g

# Roasted Brussels Sprouts

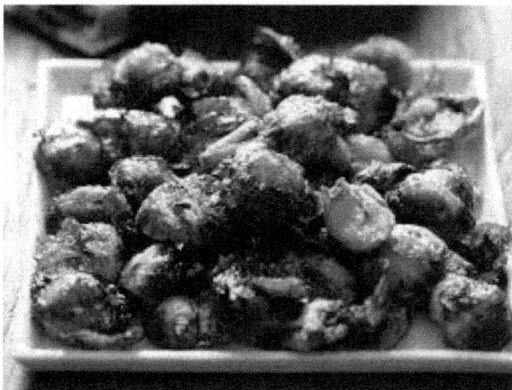

Preparation Time: 5 minutes

Cooking Time: 15 minutes

Servings: 2

**Ingredients:**

- 1 lb. Brussels sprouts
- ½ tsp. kosher salt
- 5 tsps. Olive oil

**Directions:**

1. Remove outer leaves with bruises and trim the stems. Slice vertically into 2. Rinse them and shake off excess liquid. Put them in a dish.
2. Stir in olive oil and salt to coat evenly.

3. Preheat the Air Fryer at 3900F. Arrange the prepared sprouts in the cooking basket and cook for 15 minutes.

4. Shake the basket occasionally during the cooking process.

**Nutrition:** Calories: 198 Fat: 12.4g Carbs: 20.6g Protein: 7.7g

# Air Fried Potatoes with Bell Peppers

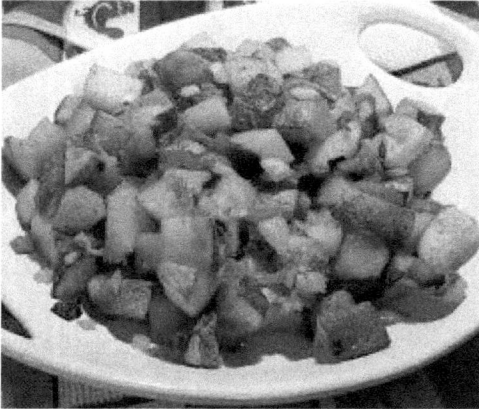

Preparation Time: 2 minutes

Cooking Time: 15 minutes

Servings: 2

**Ingredients:**

- ½ chopped onion
- 3 cubed potatoes
- 2 chopped red bell peppers
- 1 tsp. olive oil
- Salt and Black pepper

**Directions:**

1. Preheat Air Fryer at a temperature of 350°F.
2. Sprinkle salt and pepper on potatoes and drizzle olive oil toss to combine.

3. Place potatoes into fryer basket and leave to cook for 10 minutes.
4. Shake fryer basket after every 5 minutes.
5. Now add red bell peppers, onion and cook again for 5 minutes.
6. Serve.

**Nutrition** Calories: 289 Protein: 7.46 g  Fat: 2.68 g  Carbs: 61.24 g

# Air fried Stuffed Peppers

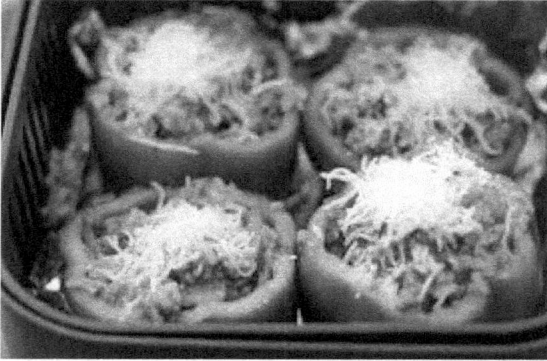

Preparation Time: 15 minutes

Cooking Time: 13 minutes

Servings: 2

**Ingredients:**

- Eggs, 4.
- Halved and deseeded bell pepper, 1.
- Salt and pepper
- Olive oil, 1 tsp.
- Sriracha flakes, ¼ tsp.

**Directions:**

1. Rub the bell pepper with olive oil around the edges.
2. Crack two eggs directly into each half of the bell pepper.
3. Drizzle all the spices over the eggs.

4. Place the included trivet in the air fryer and place the bell pepper over the trivet.
5. Close the fryer and cook the peppers on Crisper mode at 3900 F for 13 minutes then serve.

**Nutrition:** Calories: 164 Fat: 10 g Carbs: 4 g Protein: 11 g

# Garlic Cheese Bread

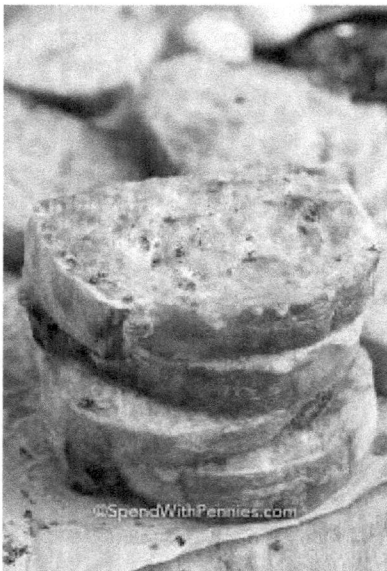

Preparation Time: 15 minutes

Cooking Time: 10 minutes

Servings: 4

**Ingredients:**

- Large egg, 1.
- Grated parmesan cheese, ¼ cup
- Garlic powder, ½ tsp.
- Shredded mozzarella cheese, 1 cup

**Directions:**

1. Layer the air fryer basket with parchment paper.

2. Mix parmesan cheese, mozzarella cheese, garlic powder, and egg in a suitable bowl.
3. Set the mixture in a well-greased pan and place this pan in the fryer basket.
4. Return the basket to the fryer.
5. Leave them to cook for 10 minutes at 3500 F on Air Fryer Mode.
6. Slice and serve warm.

**Nutrition:** Calories: 225 Fat: 14.3 g Carbs: 2.8 g Protein: 28.2 g

# Chili Cream Soufflé

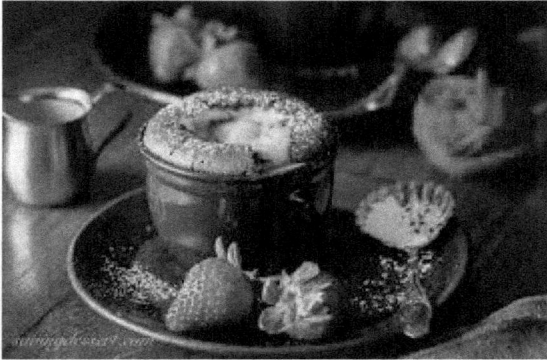

Preparation Time: 5 minutes

Cooking Time: 10 minutes

Servings: 4

**Ingredients:**

- Free-range eggs, 4.
- Large red chili pepper, ¼ tsp.
- Chopped fresh parsley.
- Cream, 4 tbsps.
- Salt and pepper.

**Directions:**

1. Preheat your air fryer to 390 °F and grease some ramekin dishes.
2. Take a large bowl and add the eggs, whisking well to combine.

3. Add the cream, parsley and chili and stir well to combine.

4. Transfer the egg mixture into the ramekin dishes up to about halfway.

5. Pop into the air fryer and cook for 10 minutes until perfect.

6. Serve and enjoy.

**Nutrition:** Calories: 127 Carbs: 3g Protein: 10g Fat: 7g

# Cheese and Bacon Breakfast Bombs

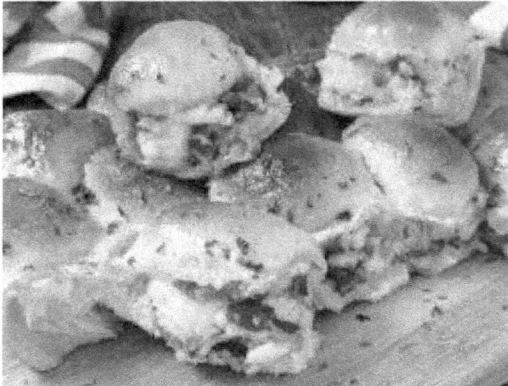

Preparation Time: 10 minutes

Cooking Time: 5 minutes

Servings: 2

**Ingredients:**

- Large eggs, 3.
- Centre-cut bacon slices, 3.
- Low carb pizza dough, 4 oz.
- Chopped fresh chives, 1 tbsp.
- Softened cream cheese, 1 oz.

**Directions:**

1. Pop a pan over medium heat and cook the bacon for ten minutes until crisp.

2. Remove from the heat and crumble, then pop to one side.
3. Stir the eggs to the pan and cook until set. Remove from the heat.
4. Place the eggs into a bowl with the cream cheese, chives and bacon.
5. Preheat your air fryer to 350°F.
6. Next take the pizza dough and carefully cut it into four pieces.
7. Roll each piece into a circle.
8. Place ¼ of the egg mixture into the middle and fold over the sides of the dough to meet in the middle.
9. Pop into the air fryer and cook for 5 minutes until perfectly cooked.

**Nutrition:** Calories: 305 Carbs: 23g Protein: 19g Fat: 15g

# LUNCH

## Juicy Pork Chops

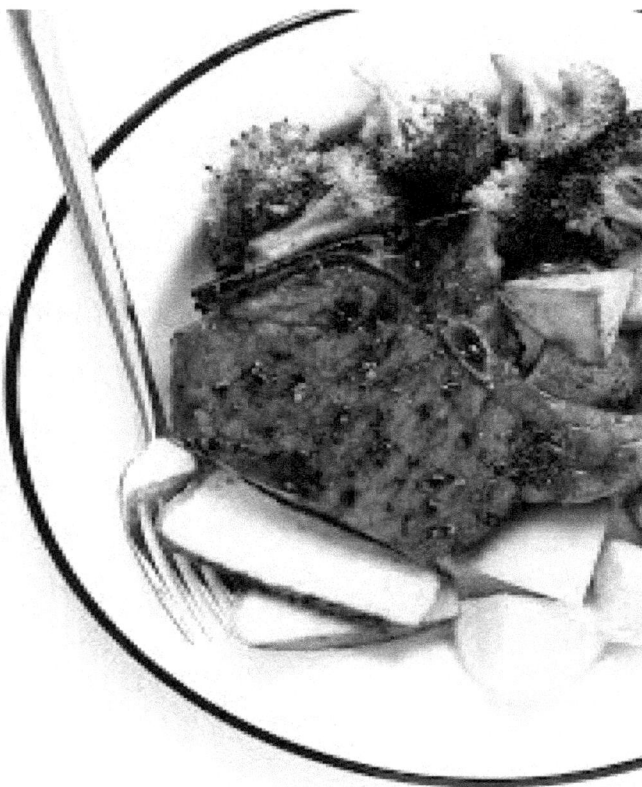

Basic Recipe

Preparation Time: 10 minutes

Cooking Time: 16 minutes

Servings: 4

**Ingredients:**

- 4 pork chops, boneless
- 2 tsp olive oil
- ½ tsp celery seed
- ½ tsp parsley
- ½ tsp granulated onion
- ½ tsp granulated garlic
- ¼ tsp sugar
- ½ tsp salt

**Directions:**

1. In a small bowl, mix together oil, celery seed, parsley, granulated onion, granulated garlic, sugar, and salt.
2. Rub seasoning mixture all over the pork chops.
3. Place pork chops on the air fryer oven pan and cook at 350 F for 8 minutes
4. Turn pork chops to other side and cook for 8 minutes more.
5. Serve and enjoy.

**Nutrition:** Calories 279 Fat 22.3 g Carbs 0.6 g Protein 18.1 g

# Crispy Meatballs

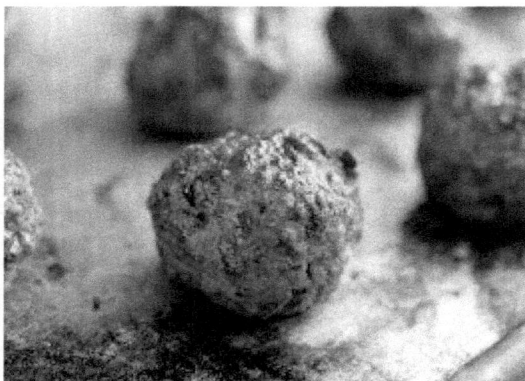

Basic Recipe

Preparation Time: 10 minutes

Cooking Time: 12 minutes

Servings: 8

**Ingredients:**

- 1 lb. ground pork
- 1 lb. ground beef
- 1 tbsp Worcestershire sauce
- ½ cup feta cheese, crumbled
- ½ cup breadcrumbs
- 2 eggs, lightly beaten
- ¼ cup fresh parsley, chopped
- 1 tbsp garlic, minced
- 1 onion, chopped
- ¼ tsp pepper

- 1 tsp salt

**Directions:**

1. Add all ingredients into the mixing bowl and mix until well combined.
2. Spray air fryer oven tray pan with cooking spray.
3. Make small balls from meat mixture and arrange on a pan and air fry t 400 F for 10-12 minutes
4. Serve and enjoy.

**Nutrition:** Calories 263 Fat 9 g Carbs 7.5 g Protein 35.9 g

# Flavorful Steak

Basic Recipe

Preparation Time: 10 minutes

Cooking Time: 18 minutes

Servings: 2

**Ingredients:**

- 2 steaks, rinsed and pat dry
- ½ tsp garlic powder
- 1 tsp olive oil
- Pepper
- Salt

**Directions:**

1. Rub steaks with olive oil and season with garlic powder, pepper, and salt.
2. Preheat the instant vortex air fryer oven to 400 F.
3. Place steaks on air fryer oven pan and air fry for 10-18 minutes turn halfway through.
4. Serve and enjoy.

**Nutrition:** Calories 361 Fat 10.9 g Carbs 0.5 g Protein 61.6 g

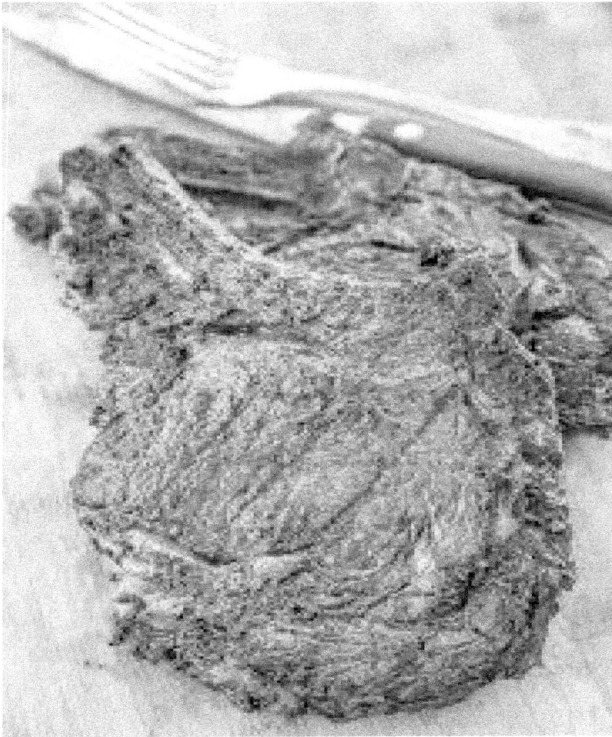

# Lemon Garlic Lamb Chops

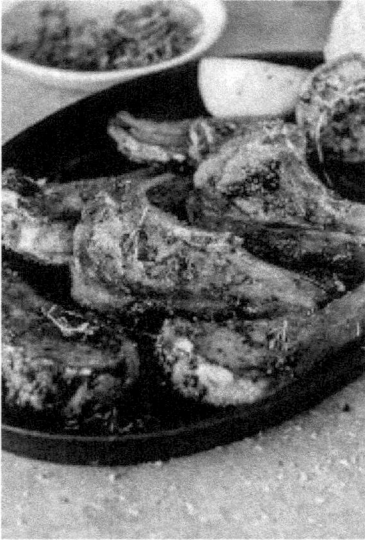

Basic Recipe

Preparation Time: 10 minutes

Cooking Time: 6 minutes

Servings: 6

**Ingredients:**

- 6 lamb loin chops
- 2 tbsp fresh lemon juice
- 1 ½ tbsp lemon zest
- 1 tbsp dried rosemary
- 1 tbsp olive oil
- 1 tbsp garlic, minced
- Pepper

- Salt

**Directions:**

1. Add lamb chops in a mixing bowl. Add remaining ingredients on top of lamb chops and coat well.
2. Arrange lamb chops on air fryer oven tray and air fry at 400 F for 3 minutes. Turn lamb chops to another side and air fry for 3 minutes more.
3. Serve and enjoy.

**Nutrition:** Calories 69 Fat 6 g Carbs 1.2 g Protein 3 g

# Easy Rosemary Lamb Chops

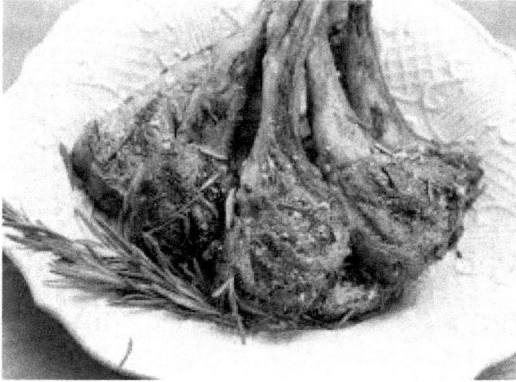

Basic Recipe

Preparation Time: 10 minutes

Cooking Time: 6 minutes

Servings: 4

**Ingredients:**

- 4 lamb chops
- 2 tbsp dried rosemary
- ¼ cup fresh lemon juice
- Pepper
- Salt

**Directions:**

1. In a small bowl, mix together lemon juice, rosemary, pepper, and salt. Brush lemon juice rosemary mixture over lamb chops.

2. Place lamb chops on air fryer oven tray and air fry at 400 F for 3 minutes. Turn lamb chops to the other side and cook for 3 minutes more. Serve and enjoy.

**Nutrition:** Calories 267 Fat 21.7 g Carbs 1.4 g Protein 16.9 g

# BBQ Pork Ribs

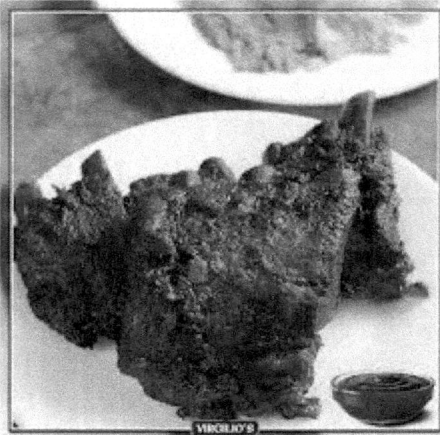

Basic Recipe

Preparation Time: 10 minutes

Cooking Time: 12 minutes

Servings: 6

**Ingredients:**

- 1 slab baby back pork ribs, cut into pieces
- ½ cup BBQ sauce
- ½ tsp paprika
- Salt

**Directions:**

1. Add pork ribs in a mixing bowl. Add BBQ sauce, paprika, and salt over pork ribs and coat well and set aside for 30 minutes

2. Preheat the instant vortex air fryer oven to 350 F. Arrange marinated pork ribs on instant vortex air fryer oven pan and cook for 10-12 minutes Turn halfway through.

3. Serve and enjoy.

**Nutrition:** Calories 145 Fat 7 g Carbs 10 g Protein 9 g

# Juicy Steak Bites

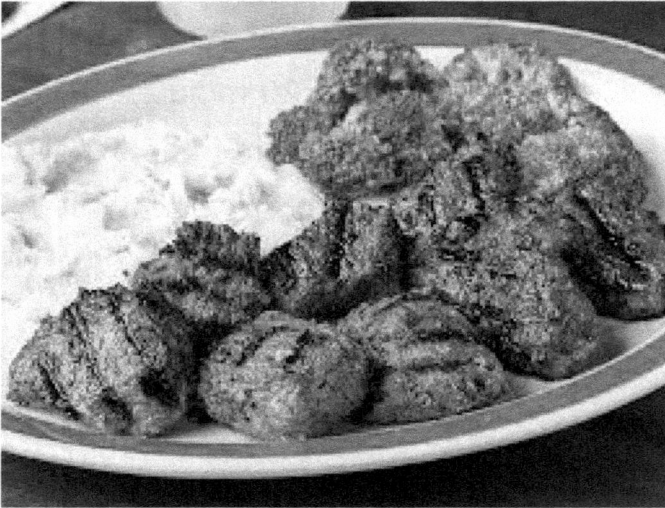

Basic Recipe

Preparation Time: 10 minutes

Cooking Time: 9 minutes

Servings: 4

**Ingredients:**

- 1 lb. sirloin steak, cut into bite-size pieces
- 1 tbsp steak seasoning
- 1 tbsp olive oil
- Pepper
- Salt

**Directions:**

1. Preheat the instant vortex air fryer oven to 390 F.

2. Add steak pieces into the large mixing bowl. Add steak seasoning, oil, pepper, and salt over steak pieces and toss until well coated.
3. Transfer steak pieces on instant vortex air fryer pan and air fry for 5 minutes
4. Turn steak pieces to the other side and cook for 4 minutes more.
5. Serve and enjoy.

**Nutrition:** Calories 241 Fat 10.6 g Carbs 0 g Protein 34.4 g

# Greek Lamb Chops

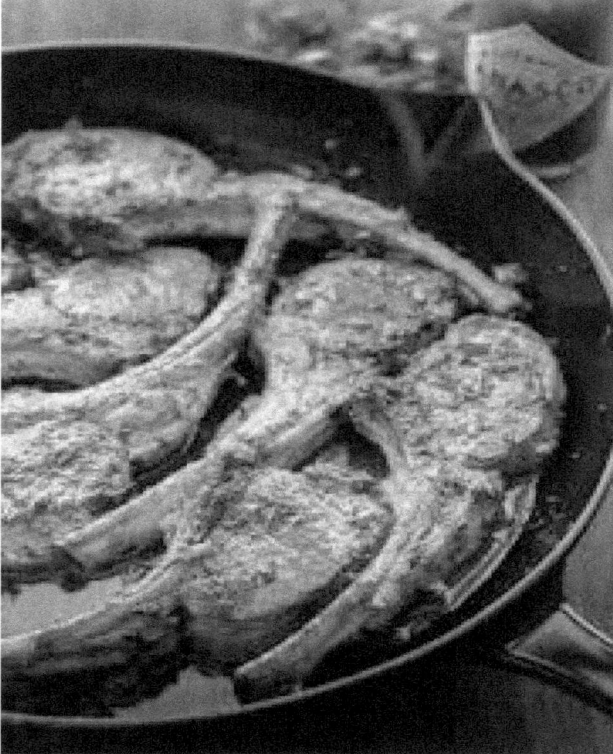

Basic Recipe

Preparation Time: 10 minutes

Cooking Time: 10 minutes

Servings: 4

**Ingredients:**

- 2 lbs. lamb chops
- 2 tsp garlic, minced
- 1 ½ tsp dried oregano

- ¼ cup fresh lemon juice
- ¼ cup olive oil
- ½ tsp pepper
- 1 tsp salt

**Directions:**

1. Add lamb chops in a mixing bowl. Add remaining ingredients over the lamb chops and coat well.
2. Arrange lamb chops on the air fryer oven tray and cook at 400 F for 5 minutes
3. Turn lamb chops and cook for 5 minutes more.
4. Serve and enjoy.

**Nutrition:** Calories 538 Fat 29.4 g Carbs 1.3 g Protein 64 g

# Easy Beef Roast

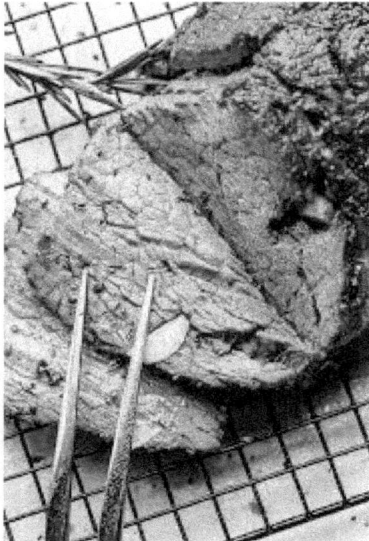

Basic Recipe

Preparation Time: 10 minutes

Cooking Time: 45 minutes

Servings: 6

**Ingredients:**

- 2 ½ lbs. beef roast
- 2 tbsp Italian seasoning

**Directions:**

1. Arrange roast on the rotisserie spite.
2. Rub roast with Italian seasoning then insert into the instant vortex air fryer oven.

3. Air fry at 350 F for 45 minutes or until the internal temperature of the roast reaches to 145 F.

4. Slice and serve.

**Nutrition:** Calories 365 Fat 13.2 g Carbs 0.5 g Protein 57.4 g

# Herb Butter Rib-eye Steak

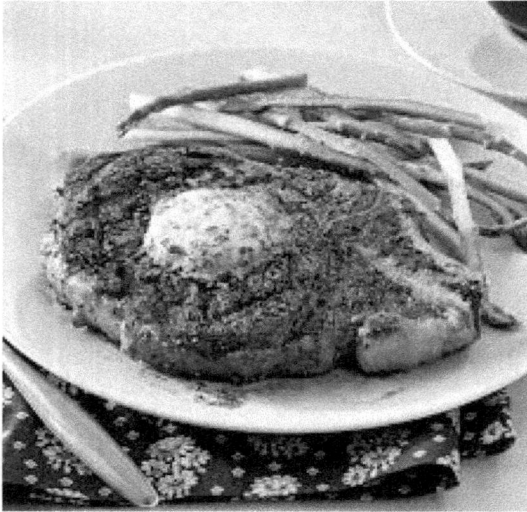

Basic Recipe

Preparation Time: 10 minutes

Cooking Time: 14 minutes

Servings: 4

**Ingredients:**

- 2 lbs. rib eye steak, bone-in
- 1 tsp fresh rosemary, chopped
- 1 tsp fresh thyme, chopped
- 1 tsp fresh chives, chopped
- 2 tsp fresh parsley, chopped
- 1 tsp garlic, minced
- ¼ cup butter softened
- Pepper

- Salt

**Directions:**

1. In a small bowl, combine together butter and herbs.
2. Rub herb butter on rib-eye steak and place it in the refrigerator for 30 minutes
3. Place marinated steak on instant vortex air fryer oven pan and cook at 400 F for 12-14 minutes
4. Serve and enjoy.

**Nutrition:** Calories 416 Fat 36.7 g Carbs 0.7 g Protein 20.3 g

# Classic Beef Jerky

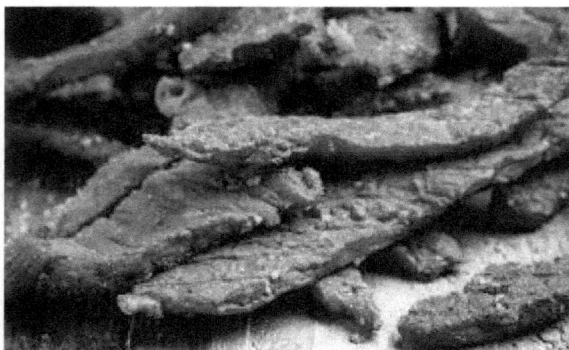

Basic Recipe

Preparation Time: 10 minutes

Cooking Time: 4 hours

Servings: 4

**Ingredients:**

- 2 lbs. London broil, sliced thinly
- 1 tsp onion powder
- 3 tbsp brown sugar
- 3 tbsp soy sauce
- 1 tsp olive oil
- 3/4 tsp garlic powder

**Directions:**

1. Add all ingredients except meat in the large zip-lock bag.
2. Mix until well combined. Add meat in the bag.

3. Seal bag and massage gently to cover the meat with marinade.

4. Let marinate the meat for 1 hour.

5. Arrange marinated meat slices on instant vortex air fryer tray and dehydrate at 160 F for 4 hours.

**Nutrition:** Calories 133 Fat 4.7 g Carbs 9.4 g Protein 13.4 g

# CONCLUSION

Air fryers are a relatively new piece of kitchen gadgetry. They are used by individuals who want to cook healthy foods using less oil and less fat then their conventional counterparts.

In addition to being a healthier alternative to deep frying, air fryers are also fun to use. Air-frying not only produces lots of fun and tasty food, it also saves you time and money. You can cook without the need of a griddle or a stovetop, which frees up your kitchen so you can focus on eating more healthy foods!

It is important to have an air fryer that is up to par. If you want an air fryer that will last for years, make sure that you buy an durable one. To help you choose the right air fryer for you, we have compiled a list of the best air fried ovens!

The Airfryer has several seating options. The four different versions include:

Small Seating–The size of the seating area is 13.5" x 8.5" x 9.5'.

Medium Seating–Tne size of the seating area is 20" x 12".

Large Seating–The size of the seating area is 23" x 15".

Extra Large Seating–The size is 32" X 21". The extra large seat could accommodate up to 8 pieces. A small, medium or large fryer is included with every air fryer and can be purchased separately. The only part that may need to be purchased separately is a colander for the basket which will hold up to 16 cups depending on the size of the basket that you are using. There are no other accessories required for the air fryer: please see the specifications on this page for further details.

What's happening to our restaurant food? The answer is rather simple. We are over-cooking and over-frying foods, and most of it is for the wrong reasons.

Nobody wants to eat overcooked, undercooked, or under-salted food. Restaurant owners are turning away good customers in the name of profit.

That's not our fault. It's up to the professional chefs to do a better job with their cooking skills.

We use our Air Fryers to cook foods that don't require cooking at all. We use them to cook and heat our foods in such a way that they're ready to eat right out of the air fryer. There's no need for you to heat up your kitchen with a conventional oven or stove, just put the food in and let it finish fully. You'll be amazed at how delicious your foods can taste when you use an Air Fryer!

Today's busy lifestyle often leaves us with little time to cook. For those of you who don't have time to cook, but still need your food, the air fryer is for you.

An air fryer is an appliance that cooks food by circulating hot air over it. The circulating air causes the food to slowly cook within a sealed container while removing excess oil and fat from the food. By sealing the food in a hermetic chamber during cooking, no additional oil is released into the air. This is important because it prevents the flavor of the food from being compromised. The result is a fast and easy way to prepare delicious meals without having to use any grease or oils while eroding your pantry of oils.

In this air fryer cookbook, we will teach you how to use your air fryer most effectively and how to avoid common mistakes. From learning how to clean and maintain your air fryer to finding creative recipes, this guide will help you get the most out of your air fryer today

CPSIA information can be obtained
at www.ICGtesting.com
Printed in the USA
BVHW091203070521
606762BV00002B/122

9 781801 838214